CHAIR YOGA FOR SENIORS, WOMEN OVER AGE 60

Serene Movement for Women 60+.
To their Elevate Well-being and
Embrace Joy.

JANIE L. DUKES

Table of content

Introduction

A group of sixty-plus senior women congregated in a quiet corner of the community center, their faces engraved with the memories of a lifetime of stories mixed with the faint strains of classical music. With the room bathed in a warm glow from the windows, they set off on a chair yoga adventure that would take them not to far-off places or historical periods but rather to a place of wellbeing and renewal.

These strong, elegant ladies were lured by the practice's charm since it promised not just physical vigor but also a comprehensive sense of well-being. It was a subdued call to embrace the flexibility that goes beyond the physique, to reclaim the strength inside, and to enjoy the peace that arises with every conscious breath and to appreciate the flexibility that goes beyond simple physicality.

The instructor's soft instruction permeated the room as they took their seats. The adventure began with a promise: to write a new chapter of vitality, to honor the stories their bodies had lived, and to bridge the gap between age and agility. This was more than simply a workout regimen; it was an embrace of a philosophy honoring age-old knowledge and the beauty that results from the harmonious dance of the body, mind, and soul.

The chair yoga practice turned into a haven where creaking joints whispered tales of resilience and laughter lines spoke to a life well-lived, all amid shared laughter and supportive nods. The teacher took them through soft warm-ups, calming stretches, and positions that unfurled like pages of a beloved novel. She was a beacon of wisdom and compassion.

Chair yoga for elderly ladies over 60 in this peaceful sanctuary evolved from a physical workout to a celebration of longevity, a tribute to life's lessons learned through experience, and a monument to the persevering spirit that sought rejuvenation. The chairs became thrones of empowerment, and these women wrote a story of elegance, courage, and the magnificent art of aging gracefully with every breath.

 And so began a trip that was motivated by their emotions rather than the passage of time, demonstrating the resilience of each person's unique life story at every turn. What was once a plain room is now a representation of a society united by the belief that old age is a blank canvas ready to be filled with life and meaningful living.

In the field of holistic health, chair yoga is gaining popularity as a personalized practice that offers senior women over 60 an amazing opportunity to begin their journey toward mindful living and physical restoration. These women gather in this serene setting, having experienced much together. to investigate the potential advantages and benefits that chair yoga offers.

Unlike traditional forms of exercise, chair yoga transcends the constraints that come with getting older. Its allure stems from its ability to provide a comprehensive sense of well-being in addition to boosting physical vigor. It becomes a practice where sitting becomes a platform for renewal and every soft movement has the capacity to bring about fresh strength, flexibility, and peace.

This trip is led by a skilled instructor and includes thoughtful breathing techniques, gentle stretches, and seated positions. Formerly a functional piece of furniture, the chair now serves as a prop for empowerment, encouraging exploration of the whole range of motion and serving as a representation of one's own potential.

Joined by a common life stage, the participants learn that chair yoga is more than just a set of poses; it's a celebration of life's lessons learned through experience, a tribute to the body's tenacity, and an appreciation of the grace that comes with growing older. Laughter blends with deliberate breathing in this area, fostering a fusion of the mental and the physical.

Chair yoga is more than just an exercise program for senior ladies over 60; it's an invitation to rediscover one's relationship with one's body and accept the subtle beauty that accompanies aging. It's a trip into the present, where every breath serves as a reminder of the enduring energy within and every movement transforms into an act of self-care. These women take a seat and begin a journey of discovery that will change them forever. It is a story of resilience, equilibrium, and the eternal spirit that go hand in hand with the skill of gracefully aging.

Purpose of Chair Yoga

Chair yoga is a deliberate practice that offers its soft embrace to a wide range of people, especially meeting the specific needs of those who are looking for the combination of accessibility and mindful movement. Its core is to promote health and well-being for people of all ages and physical capacities, going beyond what conventional yoga styles may offer.

Chair yoga's primary goal is to offer a supportive environment for people who might find it difficult to perform traditional yoga poses because of physical restrictions, age-related concerns, or mobility issues. The practice becomes inclusive when a chair is included because it enables participants to perform a variety of seated moves or to use the chair for support and balance.

This is not just an adaptation, but a demonstration of the idea that yoga is a modality that can be tailored to suit different degrees of physical ability. With chair yoga, people can re-establish a connection with their bodies and develop a sense of agency and mindfulness in each action.

Chair yoga has benefits for mental and emotional health in addition to the physical. Breathwork and movement, combined with a deliberate and attentive approach, produce a contemplative experience that provides a break from the stresses of everyday life. In between sitting poses and mild stretches, it transforms into a stress-reduction haven that encourages calmness and relaxation.

Chair yoga recognizes the connection between mind, body, and spirit, which is another way it promotes the idea of holistic wellness. It supports a better understanding of one's body and a good attitude about aging by encouraging participants to develop self-awareness.

Essentially, chair yoga aims to democratize yoga and make its many advantages available to a larger group of people. It is evidence that people of all ages and physical ailments may benefit from the transforming power of yoga, demonstrating the flexibility and inclusion ingrained in the age-old practice. This practice becomes a vehicle for empowerment, self-discovery, and a path towards total well-being through the humble chair.

Benefits for Senior Women

As a specially designed practice for senior women, chair yoga offers a multitude of advantages that transcend well beyond the sphere of the body. It functions as a haven where these ladies can investigate the symbiotic fusion of body, mind, and soul.

Chair yoga becomes a soft ally in terms of the body, encouraging mobility and flexibility without putting the body through excessive strain. It provides a break for bodies that have withstood the test of time by easing muscular tension and promoting joint health through deliberate stretches and motions.

However, its impact extends beyond the physical realm. Senior women who practice chair yoga are invited to be fully present in the moment as it unfolds, thus serving as a conduit for the cultivation of mindfulness. It provides a meditative place through the rhythmic ebb and flow of breath and movement, promoting emotional balance and cerebral clarity.

Adopting the inclusion idea, chair yoga transforms into a wellness industry democratizer. It respects each participant's individuality by letting them interact with the practice at their own speed and in accordance with their particular physical capabilities. Senior women who possess this flexibility feel more empowered, since it gives them control over their bodies and enhances their positive self-image.

Beyond the obvious mental and physical benefits, chair yoga fosters a sense of belonging. These women find companionship in their common practice, where they exchange stories, laughs, and the collective wisdom of their individual experiences. The chair, which was formerly just a seat, becomes a communal area where coordinated breathing and movement create a fabric of shared wellbeing.

In essence, chair yoga transforms into a kind mentorship that invites older ladies to accept the beauty that comes with growing older, to savor the richness of the present, and to recognize the resiliency of their bodies. This technique becomes a vehicle for empowerment, promoting a comprehensive sense of well-being that goes beyond the constraints frequently associated with aging, all through the modest support of a chair. Through the cultivation of a comprehensive feeling of well-being that transcends the constraints frequently associated with aging, this practice becomes a vehicle for empowerment. Chair yoga transforms from a physical workout into a celebration of the elegance and tenacity that characterize the extraordinary journey of senior women as it moves between sitting poses and focused breathing.

Getting Started

Taking up chair yoga for older ladies is like accepting an invitation to a voyage of focused discovery and gradual blossoming, which starts with accepting the present moment. Recognizing this practice's distinctiveness is the first step towards creating an inclusive haven where age is not a barrier but rather a blank canvas for revitalized energy.

Selecting the ideal chair becomes essential, serving not only as a practical seat but also as a guide on this life-changing adventure. Choosing a chair that is comfy, firm, and has a straight back without armrests promotes stability and gives you confidence to perform each activity.

The senior women acknowledge their safety as they take their seats in this particular chair to begin the exercise. The voyage begins with mild stretches of the neck, a gentle preamble to the symphony of movement that unfolds. These first motions act as a link between the body's consciousness and the breathing's regular rhythm.

The warm-up stage transforms into a gentle ritual of motions intended to arouse the body. Shoulder rolls become a dance, releasing stored tension in the upper body, and cat-cow stretches while seated create a dialogue between the spine and the breath that promotes flexibility with each flowing movement.

Asanas, or seated positions, are the core of the exercise. As an affirmation of grounding and a link to the earth below, mountain pose emerges. Bends that are seated forward promote giving in to the present moment, a soft stretch that extends past the body into the domain of reflection.

As the voyage continues through sequences created for different times of the day, the chair changes into a prop for stability. Morning rituals bring in a feeling of renewal; afternoon exercises provide opportunities for relaxation; and evening wind-downs turn into a ritual of thanksgiving, a group recognition of the day's work.

Chair yoga incorporates breathing methods, which are a subtle but effective addition. By engaging in a rhythmic dance with the breath, diaphragmatic breathing helps cultivate a connection to the life force inside. Breathing via alternate nostrils can become a meditative exercise that promotes calm and equilibrium.

Chair yoga for senior ladies goes beyond the physical poses and explores stability and balance. A sense of groundedness is fostered in every moment by heel and toe taps, and seated leg lifts turn into a celebration of power.

Seated leg stretches and ankle rolls are examples of flexibility exercises that encourage participants to fully explore their range of motion and serve as a gentle reminder of their innate suppleness.

The cool-down and relaxation phases begin as the chair transforms into a tool for movement and reflection. With attentive breathing providing a calming rhythm and guided relaxation turning into a contemplative experience, the women are able to savor the aftereffects of their practice.

At its peak, chair yoga for older ladies goes beyond the basic physical aspect of fitness. It turns into a story, a tale of deliberate movement, deliberate breathing, and a subdued celebration of the beauty, resiliency, and strength that come with growing older with grace and energy.

Safety Precautions

As elderly women embrace chair yoga—a practice meant to celebrate their individual path of aging with grace and vitality—it is imperative to create a secure and supportive environment. The practice incorporates safety considerations smoothly, laying the groundwork for each participant to begin their journey of conscious movement and self-discovery.

Selecting a good chair turns out to be the first line of defense—more than just a place to sit. A strong chair without armrests and a straight back provides a stable base so that the woman can confidently explore the exercise. Setting up the chair on a non-slip surface strengthens its base even more and guarantees stability with every motion.

In chair yoga, safety is based on the recognition of each practitioner's unique demands and physical state. As they embrace the self-awareness that leads them through the exercise, participants are urged to listen to their bodies. Adjustments turn into a kind partner, providing versions of every motion to suit different degrees of comfort and flexibility.

Establishing a safe environment is the duty of the instructor, a guiding force on this path. Gentle and unambiguous verbal signals turn into a navigational aid, directing the women through every move with accuracy. By keeping an eye on things closely, the instructor may make tailored corrections that help every student feel safe and supported while they explore.

Promoting a slow and steady tempo among participants cultivates a secure atmosphere. The focus is on accepting one's own breathing rhythm and the distinct cadence of one's body's reaction to movement, not on pushing boundaries. Being patient becomes a defensive strategy that enables every woman to enjoy the adventure as it unfolds without rushing.

Being aware of any prior injuries or medical issues becomes essential to your safety. Open communication between participants and the instructor is encouraged in order to provide pertinent information that helps tailor the practice to each participant's needs. By creating a bridge through this open communication, the practice is guaranteed to continue being a source of support rather than stress.

The instructor encourages the elderly women to use props or extra assistance as needed as they get more comfortable with the activity. This could incorporate blocks for stability or cushions for enhanced comfort. As allies, these items improve the experience and add to the overall feeling of security.

The instructor stays sensitive to the participants' emotional health in the spirit of holistic safety. A positive environment is created by affirmations and gentle encouragement, which strengthen the bond between the mind, body, and spirit and promote a sense of success.

As a result of these safety measures, chair yoga for older women develops into a sanctuary where the entwining strands of support, awareness, and self-kindness create a tapestry of wellbeing rather than just a physical workout. By taking these deliberate steps, the practice transforms into a celebration of fortitude, resiliency, and the eternal spirit, which go hand in hand with the skill of aging with grace.

Choosing the Right Chair

A careful and crucial first step in practicing chair yoga is choosing the right chair, which will match the physical support to the particular requirements of senior ladies over 60. This decision goes beyond simple use, making the chair a reliable travel companion for mindful movement and overall well being.

The perfect chair has characteristics that enhance comfort and stability. Being sturdy makes the chair a vital requirement, guaranteeing that it offers a stable base for a range of motions. A straight-backed chair provides essential support for appropriate alignment in seated poses, promoting the sensation of stability that is the foundation of the practice.

Even though they are frequently linked to comfort, armrests are taken into account when practicing chair yoga. Choosing a chair with no armrests increases range of motion and makes it easier to strike a variety of positions. This design decision allows participants to freely explore the practice's potential through unrestricted gestures.

In order to guarantee that the feet can rest comfortably flat on the floor, seat height is important. This arrangement promotes stability and balance during seated poses and mild motions. The chair serves as an extension of the ground, providing the older women with a stable foundation on which to confidently engage in the exercise.

The overall comfort of the chair is enhanced by careful consideration of the seat material. Long durations of sitting are made more comfortable and easeful for participants thanks to the soothing surface provided by a cushioned seat. With this well-considered addition, the chair becomes a place of support and comfort.

The chair's dimensions are important in relation to each participant's unique needs. Adequate breadth and depth of chairs facilitate a variety of body types, guaranteeing that every woman may comfortably sink into the chair with sufficient space for mobility. This diversity serves as evidence of chair yoga's individualized approach.

During the practice, it is safer to place the chair on a non-slip surface. By taking this precaution, the chair won't accidentally move and will stay steady when the women change into different stances. As a result, stability becomes crucial for safe mobility exploration without the fear of slipping.

In the end, the chair used for chair yoga serves as a silent companion on the path to wellbeing, rather than just a prop. It turns into a symbol of the practice's versatility, a source of support, and a way to facilitate mobility. A harmonic and enriching experience is created when senior ladies over 60 carefully choose the perfect chair, one that is personalized to their needs and can become a conduit for thoughtful exploration, strength, and graceful aging.

Warm-Up Exercises

The practice of chair yoga for women over 60 begins with a gentle warm-up intended to awaken the body and develop an awareness of the relationship between breath and movement. This stage provides a calm beginning, encouraging a feeling of comfort and readiness for the practice's evolving path.

Gentle neck stretches are a graceful way to start the warm-up. They are a rhythmic conversation between the head and the neck, a preamble that helps release tension held in these sensitive areas. Seated in their preferred seats, the women move slowly and deliberately, encouraging a nuanced examination of movement.

The last traces of stiffness are swept away by the flowing waltz of shoulder rolls. The seated participants discover a rhythm that goes beyond the physical as the shoulders elegantly revolve; the flowing motion becomes a metaphorical release of responsibilities, opening the door for a lighter, more liberated connection with the exercise.

Cat-cow stretches while seated create a symphony of breath and spine. The women invite the spine to curve in a wave-like motion by articulating the movements at a slow, deliberate speed. The relationship between breath and movement in this choreography is tangible; it's a dance that transcends the physical into the domain of attentive awareness.

Every warm-up turns into a gentle investigation—a call to recognize the body's own rhythm and cultivate awareness of the present moment. The chair, a silent observer of these motions, becomes a support structure that gives the senior women a firm base from which to launch the practice.

There's a gradual waking that permeates the entire organism, and the warmth generated during these first movements transcends the physical. The warm-up evolves from a set of exercises into a ritual, a ceremony that signifies the change from stillness to deliberate movement and from a routine self-care practice to an exceptional one.

The warm-up activities in chair yoga for older women serve as a gentle introduction to the practice, allowing participants to enter a state of wellbeing and self-discovery. It's a gentle introduction, a recognition that every breath and action has the capacity to bring about a resurgence of energy and a closer relationship with the body's innate understanding. The women begin to experience a journey that goes beyond time limitations as they become accustomed to the pace of the warm-up. This journey invites them to appreciate the beauty of movement, breath, and the delicate art of aging with grace.

Gentle Neck Stretches

Chair yoga for senior ladies over 60 uses slow, deliberate motions to enhance flexibility and release tension in the neck. Start by taking a comfortable seat in a chair and keeping your back straight. As you exhale, gently tilt your head to one side with the intention of bringing your ear closer to your shoulder. Take a deep breath, lengthening your spine. Feel the stretch along the side of your neck while you hold it for a few breaths.

Go back to the center and do the opposite side. After that, take a breath and slowly tilt your head forward, bringing your chin closer to your chest as you exhale. Sensation: the strain running down the back of your neck.

After a few breaths of holding, move back to the center.

Breathe in, move your head to one side, and position your chin against your shoulder to extend the other side of your neck. Feel the soft release as you hold the stretch. Repeat on the other side, then inhale back to the center.

Lastly, make sure to include mild neck rotations. Take a big breath in, then slowly move your head to the side while holding it there for a little while. Returning your breath to the center, exhale as you rotate to the opposite side. These flowing movements lessen stiffness and increase neck mobility.

Recall to move cautiously and to stay away from any sudden or excruciating discomfort. Senior ladies over 60 can benefit from including these mild stretches into their daily routine to improve their general well-being and encourage relaxation.

Shoulder Rolls

For elderly ladies over 60, shoulder rolls in chair yoga are a great way to relieve stress and improve shoulder mobility. First, take a comfortable chair seat and make sure your feet are flat on the floor and your spine is straight. Breathe deeply and let your shoulders drop for a moment.

As you inhale, raise both shoulders toward your ears to begin the shoulder roll. Roll your shoulders back and down in a smooth, circular motion as you release your breath. Sensate the mild strain on your shoulders and upper back. For a few breaths, keep rotating while maintaining a smooth and controlled motion.

After a few rolls in the opposite direction, change course. Breathe in as you raise your shoulders and out as you lower and return them. This forward rotation encourages a well-rounded release by focusing on various shoulder and upper back muscles.

You can add changes to the stretch to make it more profound. Engage your arms in the movement by extending them out to the sides or even overhead as your shoulders roll back. This stretches the entire shoulder girdle and adds another dimension.

Keep an eye on your breathing during the shoulder rolls, taking a breath as you raise and a release as you descend. The effects of the exercise for relaxation are increased by this coordination of breath and movement. Encourage a regulated, modest tempo that will allow the joints to mobilize and the muscles to progressively release.

Shoulder rolls can be incorporated into a chair yoga practice on a regular basis to help senior ladies over 60 become more flexible, less stiff, and more relaxed. Consistent practice can help with general wellbeing and better posture.

Seated Cat-Cow Stretch

Senior ladies over 60 who practice chair yoga can relieve tension in their shoulders and upper back with ease by using shoulder rolls. First, take a comfortable chair seat and make sure your feet are flat on the floor and your spine is straight. Take a few deep breaths to center yourself for a bit.

As you take a breath, raise your shoulders toward your ears to start the shoulder rolls. Notice how the upper trapezius muscles are somewhat tense. Exhale and pull your shoulders down and towards your back by rolling them back in a circular motion. Your back should move smoothly and deliberately as your shoulder blades move over it.

Continue rotating in a circular motion, emphasizing the seamless transition between the shoulder rolls. Your shoulders should come back up to your ears when you inhale and back down when you exhale. This motion, which is repeated, improves blood flow to the shoulder area and promotes flexibility in the surrounding muscles.After a few repetitions, switch up the shoulder rolls' direction. Inhale as you bring your shoulders down to your sides, and release as you bring them up to your ears. This backward movement helps to reduce tension completely by activating many muscle fibers.

Remain mindful of your breath and in the present moment during the entire exercise. Shoulder rolls are a mild stretch that may be readily introduced into everyday routines to improve mobility and relieve stiffness in the upper back and shoulders. This makes them accessible to older ladies.

Seated Asanas (Poses)

For women over 60, chair yoga poses are an excellent way to increase your flexibility and sense of serenity. First, sit comfortably on a chair with your feet flat on the floor. Make sure your spine is aligned. Starting from a sitting position, begin with a simple twist: inhale deeply, then slowly turn your torso to one side, resting your weight with one hand on the back of the chair and the other on the knee across from you. Hold the twist for a few breaths, feeling the tension release and a slight stretch down your spine.To make a seated forward bend, take a breath and extend your spine. Then release the breath as you stretch forward and bend at the hips. Obtain or locate Feel a light stretch in your hamstrings and lower back as you extend your arms toward the floor or your thighs.

Put your hands on your knees and perform a seated cat-cow stretch. Breathe in while arching your back and raising your chest (the cow posture); as you release the breath, round your back and bring your chin to your chest (the cat position). Breathe in rhythm with the movement as you alternate between these two postures.

Investigate a seated hip opener by forming a figure-four with one ankle crossed over the other knee. To open the hip, apply light pressure to the crossed knee. After a few breaths of holding, move to the opposite side.

Finish with a relaxation or meditation position in which you sit, close your eyes, and concentrate on your breathing. Let the chair support you while you discover peace and quiet.

For senior women over 60, these seated asanas offer a moderate and approachable method to add yoga to their daily practice, fostering flexibility, balance, and overall well being.

Mountain Pose

Mountain Pose is a basic yoga stance that may be elegantly modified for chair yoga, which is helpful and accessible for elderly ladies over sixty. First, take a comfortable seat in a sturdy chair and place your feet firmly on the floor. Establish a connection with the soil underneath you.

Stretch your back while keeping your head's crown slightly up. As you find a comfortable hand position—perhaps resting them on your thighs or holding them in your lap—let your shoulders drop. Gently engage your core to promote stability.

Visualize your physique as a sturdy, rooted mountain. As you inhale deeply with your nose, fill your lungs, and gently exhale through your mouth, pay attention to your breath. Let your breathing be a steady, regular flow to help you relax.

Feel how your body is positioned, with your heart above your pelvis and your head above your heart. Accept an openness in your chest that will enhance your physical and mental health. Reduce your eye contact to promote calmness.

As you hold the Mountain Pose, acknowledge the stability and power it provides and work to create a beautiful harmony between ease and strength. Seniors can benefit from the grounding effects of Mountain Pose in a sitting adaptation that honors their individual needs and talents.

Seated Forward Bend

For elderly ladies over sixty, incorporating the Seated Forward Bend into chair yoga can offer a mild stretch that encourages flexibility and relaxation. First, take a comfortable chair seat and make sure your feet are firmly planted on the floor.

Spend a moment centering yourself and establishing a sense of physical contact with the chair. For stability, sit up straight, elongating your spine, and slightly contract your core. Breathe in deeply, pushing through your head's crown, and out slowly, letting your shoulders relax.

Lead with your chest and hinge at the hips as you begin the forward bend.

Depending on how comfortable it is for you, extend your arms forward or downward. Pay attention to your body's natural range of motion and proceed cautiously, taking your time.

Sensately extend your lower back, hamstrings, and spine. Let your neck unwind as you keep your eyes softly closed or open if it's more comfortable. Breathe slowly, allowing each exhale to relieve tension and take you a little bit more into the pose.

Accept the feelings in your body and make a connection with your breathing to promote peace and surrender. The benefits of the traditional yoga pose are provided by a seated forward bend in a chair, which also enhances flexibility and delivers a rejuvenating experience tailored to the specific needs of seniors.

Gentle Twist

Chair yoga with a gentle twist can offer a wonderful sensation of rebirth and mobility for women over 60. To begin, take a comfortable seat in your chair with your back straight and your feet flat on the ground. Take a moment to center yourself by paying attention to your breathing.As you start the twist, carefully rotate your torso to one side, using the back of the chair as support. Place one hand on the knee of the person opposite you and the other on the chair's back. Breathe out to lengthen your spine, and then begin the twist from your waist, moving your head and eyes as you do so.

Emphasize the opening through your chest and the stretch along your back as you feel the slight rotation of your spine. Move within a comfortable range while keeping an eye out for any restrictions. To enhance stability and support the twist, gently engage your core.

Breathe fluidly and steadily, allowing each breath to slightly lengthen your spine and each exhale to slightly deepen the twist. Savor the feeling of your spine becoming more supple and free of stress. Continue the twist slowly and deliberately on the opposite side.

Chair Yoga Sequences

Creating a chair yoga routine for ladies over sixty requires blending calming, strong, and flexible moves. Place your feet level on the floor, sit comfortably, and maintain a tall spine to begin. Start by taking a few deep, deliberate breaths to center yourself. To extend your neck and shoulders, gently tilt your head side to side, forward and backward. Encourage a wide range of motion.

To release tension, raise your shoulders near your ears and roll them back and forth in a smooth, circular motion. Breathe in as you raise your chest and arch your back (Cow); exhale as you tuck your chin in a seated cat-cow stretch and round your spine (Cat). To increase spine flexibility, perform these movements fluidly.

 For a seated forward bend, hinge at the hips. Reach forward while maintaining a straight spine to feel your hamstrings and back gently stretched. Hold while progressively deepening the stretch for a few breaths. With the chair's back providing support, gently shift your torso to one side. Breathe into the twist while holding onto the chair with one hand and the opposing knee with the other. Repeat on the other side. To create a sense of foundation and elevation, ground your feet into chair mountain pose, stretch your spine, and reach your arms overhead.

Stretch one leg forward while keeping the other foot planted to create a seated warrior position. As you maintain the stretch on either side, switch sides and extend your arms overhead to create a side stretch. To improve circulation, lift and rotate your ankles for ankle rolls. You may also lightly activate your leg muscles by tapping your toes on the floor. After a brief period of seated meditation, participants are encouraged to concentrate on their breathing exercises to promote mental clarity and relaxation. The goal of this chair yoga sequence is to improve the mobility, flexibility, and overall well-being of women over 60 by emphasizing gentle, flowing movements. It is suggested for participants to proceed at their own pace while honoring the requirements and limitations of their bodies.

Morning Routine

A morning chair yoga practice is a calm and invigorating approach for elderly women over sixty to start their day. First, take a seat that is comfortable and supportive in a chair, firmly plant your feet, and arch your back. For a little while, practice conscious breathing. This entails inhaling deeply with your nose and exhaling slowly through your lips.Start with simple neck stretches, which involve turning your head in different directions, to reduce tension and increase flexibility. Proceed to shoulder rolls, rising and lowering them while allowing the tension to be released by the circular motion.

Take a seat and perform a cat-cow stretch. Inhale as you raise your chest and arch your back; exhale as you turn your spine and tuck your chin. As you proceed through these exercises, your spine will become more aware and flexible.

Maintain a straight spine while bending forward from a seated position, bending at the hips. Appreciate the gradual release of tension as your hamstrings and back feel gently stretched.

Include a seated twist by turning your torso to one side softly and supporting yourself with the chair's back. Breathe into the gradual rotation while holding the twist, and then repeat on the opposite side.

As you extend your spine, ground your feet, and raise your arms aloft, go into a seated mountain posture. Accept the feeling of support and elevation that this stance offers.

 Explore a seated warrior pose by extending one leg forward and keeping the other foot fixed. For a side stretch, raise your arms above your head. As you flip sides, keep stretching on each side.To improve circulation, lift and twist your ankles. To strengthen your leg muscles, lightly tap the tips of your toes on the floor. Ankle rolls and toe taps are the names of these workouts.

After your morning ritual, spend a few minutes sitting in meditation to promote calmness and mental clarity. Pay attention to your breath, letting each inhale bring you energy and each exhalation let go of any last bits of tension.

For senior women over 60, this chair yoga sequence is meant to gently awaken the body, improve flexibility, and cultivate a good mindset first thing in the morning. While moving at their own pace and paying attention to their bodies, participants are urged to take advantage of this mindful morning practice's rejuvenating effects.

Afternoon Relaxation

For elderly ladies over sixty, an afternoon chair yoga class can be a calming and restorative respite. First, take a seat comfortably in a firm chair with your hands resting on your thighs or on your lap and your feet resting on the ground. Spend a few seconds focusing on your breathing, taking deep breaths through your nose and taking slow, deliberate exhalations through your mouth to help you relax.

To alleviate any stress that has built up throughout the day, begin with mild neck stretches by rotating your head. Promote mindfulness and the practice of being totally present during every action. As you elevate your shoulders toward your ears and roll them back and down, engage in shoulder rolls. Allow a wave of ease to sweep over you as you notice the subtle release of tension in your upper back and shoulders.

Take a seat and perform a cat-cow stretch. Inhale as you raise your chest and arch your back; exhale as you turn your spine and tuck your chin. Permit these movements' fluidity to encourage ease and flexibility.

Bend forward while seated, extending your torso forward while maintaining a straight back. Pay attention to your back lengthening and your hamstrings gently stretching. Accept the feeling of letting go and giving yourself over to the here and now.

Include a seated twist by turning your torso to one side softly and supporting yourself with the chair's back. Breathe into the gradual rotation while holding the twist, and then repeat the technique on the opposite side.

As you move into a seated mountain pose, stretch your spine and plant your feet firmly. In order to promote steadiness and serenity, raise your arms above your head.

Explore a seated warrior pose by extending one leg forward and keeping the other foot fixed. For a side stretch, raise your arms above your head.

As you flip sides, keep stretching on each side.Ankle rolls and toe taps are the final exercises. To improve circulation, lift and twist your ankles. To strengthen your leg muscles, lightly tap the tips of your toes on the floor.

Spend a few minutes at a time in seated meditation to allow your mind to relax and reach a calm condition. Appreciate the rejuvenating effects of this afternoon chair yoga practice as you pay attention to your breath.

This afternoon routine is intended to help senior ladies over 60 develop a sense of well-being, relieve tension, and foster relaxation. It is recommended that practitioners move slowly, appreciating every second and basking in the peace that chair yoga may provide.

An evening chair yoga practice can offer older women over 60 a quiet and soothing approach to winding down as the day draws to an end. Sit comfortably in a firm chair with your hands resting on your thighs or on your lap and your feet resting on the ground. Shut your eyes and spend a few minutes focusing on your breathing, taking deep breaths through your nose and gentle exhalations through your mouth to help you achieve a state of calm.

Stretch your neck slowly and deliberately at the beginning of the workout, rotating your head in different directions to relieve any residual tension. Promote a mindful presence while relishing the chance to let go of the day's worries.

As you raise your shoulders toward your ears and roll them back and forth, transition into shoulder rolls. Accept the sensation of relaxation as you feel the tension in your upper back and shoulders gently release.

Take a seat and perform a cat-cow stretch. Inhale as you raise your chest and arch your back; exhale as you turn your spine and tuck your chin. Let a feeling of ease and flexibility be fostered by the flow of these movements.

Bend forward while seated, extending your torso forward while maintaining a straight back. Let go of any pent-up tension as you concentrate on the mild stretch along your hamstrings and back.

Include a seated twist by turning your torso to one side softly and supporting yourself with the chair's back. Breathe deeply into the mild rotation while holding the twist, and then repeat the technique on the opposite side.

As you move into a seated mountain pose, stretch your spine and plant your feet firmly. Extend your arms above yourself, creating a calm and steady feeling.

Explore a seated warrior pose by extending one leg forward and keeping the other foot fixed. For a side stretch, raise your arms above your head. As you flip sides, keep stretching on each side.End the nighttime workout with ankle rolls and toe taps. To improve blood flow, lift and twist your ankles. To strengthen your leg muscles, lightly tap your toes on the ground.

Finally, take a few minutes to sit in meditation, letting your body and mind both completely rest. Pay attention to your breathing while enjoying the calm that chair yoga can provide for your nightly wind-down.

This sequence is intended to help elderly ladies over 60 develop a sense of peace, reduce stress, and nurture relaxation in the evening. Before going to bed, participants are urged to move mindfully, respecting their breathing patterns and letting chair yoga's calming effects lead them into a calm frame of mind.

Breathing Techniques

Chair yoga for older ladies over 60 can be improved by adding mindful breathing methods, which will encourage relaxation and a sense of well-being. First, take a seat comfortably in a firm chair with your hands resting on your thighs or on your lap and your feet resting on the ground.

1. Deep Abdominal Breathing: Start by breathing deeply in your abdomen. Breathe deeply through your nose, letting your diaphragm expand completely, and then gently release the breath through your mouth, emphasizing a full and gentle expiration. With every breath, feel the rise and fall of your abdomen, which will help you to relax.

2. Equal Breathing (Sama Vritti): To practice equal breathing, count to four while inhaling and outhaling. This method of breathing deeply and steadily promotes equilibrium and calmness. You can progressively increase the count for a deeper breathing sensation as you get more at ease.

3. Ujjayi Breathing, or Ocean Breath: Explain Ujjayi breathing, which is frequently referred to as the ocean Breath. Breathe in through your nose while slightly tightening the back of your throat to produce a faint oceanic sound. Breathe out using the same little restriction. This method can help you become more focused and relaxed by adding a contemplative element to your practice.

4. Alternate Nostril Breathing: Learn how to keep your equilibrium by investigating this method (Nadi Shodhana). Using your right thumb and ring finger, gently close one nostril while taking a breath in through the other. Next, close the other nostril with your thumb and release the air through the open nostril. Continue the alternating pattern to promote awareness and balance.

5. Employ the 4-7-8 Breathing Method: Use this method of breathing. Take a gentle four-count breath with your nose, hold it for seven counts, and then exhale loudly for eight counts through your mouth. This method encourages deep relaxation and stress reduction.

6. Sighing Breath: Use this technique by inhaling deeply with your nose and letting out a loud sigh as you exhale through your mouth. This eases the stress and encourages letting go.

7. Practice box breathing (also known as square breathing) by taking a breath, holding it, letting it out, and stopping for the same number of counts. Imagine the breath as a square, with each side contributing to the formation of a peaceful and balanced shape.

Stress the value of taking slow, even breaths while practicing these exercises, and encourage older women to experiment until they discover the rhythm that feels most comfortable for them. Intentional breathing combined with chair yoga can strengthen the mind-body connection and promote a more relaxed and well-rounded experience.

Diaphragmatic Breathing

For older women over sixty, chair yoga can be a simple yet powerful practice that incorporates diaphragmatic breathing, commonly known as deep belly breathing. The diaphragm is the primary breathing muscle employed in this method. The benefits of chair yoga for both physical and emotional well-being are numerous.

Starting Position: Place your feet firmly on the floor and sit comfortably on a sturdy chair. Put your hands on your thighs or in your lap to encourage a natural splaying of your spine.

Awareness: Recognize the natural rhythm of your breathing. Observe how your chest and abdomen rise with each breath and descend slightly with each release. With one hand on your chest and the other on your abdomen, start diaphragmatic breathing. Take a deep breath through your nose and push the air through your diaphragm. When your tummy rises, your lower hand expands outward, while the hand on your chest essentially stays stationary. As you gently and completely exhale via your lips or nose, let your belly naturally sink. To promote a feeling of release and relaxation, emphasize the exhalation.

Maintaining a careful awareness of the breath's travel, continue this diaphragmatic breathing rhythm. Prioritize establishing a peaceful and present atmosphere while establishing a fluid and steady flow.

Advantages:

1. Stress Reduction: By triggering the body's relaxation response, diaphragmatic breathing aids in lowering tension and anxiety.

2. Better Oxygenation: By using the diaphragm, you can increase the body's oxygenation by improving the lung's oxygen exchange efficiency.

3. Enhanced Lung Capacity: By encouraging a full breath, this method enhances respiratory health and lung capacity.

4. Circulation: Deep belly breathing has a beneficial effect on circulation, facilitating the flow of blood that is oxygenated to different body areas.

5. Posture: By using diaphragmatic breathing exercises while seated, one can become more conscious of one's posture and improve general spinal health.

Mind-Body Connection: Use diaphragmatic breathing to help senior women develop a stronger mind-body connection. Stress the practice's nourishing and restorative properties and encourage people to incorporate it into their everyday lives, as well as chair yoga sessions.

Chair yoga that incorporates diaphragmatic breathing allows older women to connect with their body's inherent rhythm, promoting mindfulness, relaxation, and overall well-being.

Alternate Nostril Breathing

Nadi Shodhana, also known as Alternate Nostril Breathing, is a pranayama (breath control) method that may be expertly modified for chair yoga, providing elderly women over 60 with a balancing and tranquil experience. By inhaling through one nostril at a time, this technique encourages a balanced flow of energy throughout the body.

Starting Position: Take a seat in a firm chair that seems comfortable for you to start. Let your spine naturally stretch by resting your hands on your thighs or in your lap. Make sure your posture is comfortable and your shoulders are relaxed.

Hand Position: Gently seal off your right nostril with your thumb. As an alternative, you can seal off your nostrils with your thumb and ring finger so that the other fingers lie on your forehead.

Breathing Pattern: 1. Take a gentle breath in through your left nostril, making sure your breathing is steady and smooth.2. Release the right nostril and use your ring finger to close the left nostril.3. Release all the air via your right nostril, gently and thoroughly.4. Breathe using your right nose.5. Shut your right nostril while opening your left.6. Gently and thoroughly exhale through your left nostril.

Repeat: For a few rounds, keep going in this manner, switching between the nostrils. Promote a leisurely, unhurried pace where the movement is guided by the breath.

Awareness: Focus on the inhalation and exhalation of each breath as it passes through each nostril. As you move between the nostrils, pay attention to any minor sensations or shifts in energy.

Advantages:

1. Balancing Energy Channels: Nadi Shodhana is thought to help maintain homeostasis by balancing the body's energy channels.

2. Soothing the Nervous System: This technique helps to lower tension and anxiety by soothing the nervous system.

3. Improving Focus: Alternate Nostril Breathing is a gentle yet efficient method of bringing the mind into balance. It is believed to improve focus and mental clarity.

4. Better Respiratory Function: This method can improve lung capacity and respiratory function by deliberately controlling the breath via each nostril.

5. Mind-Body Connection: To promote inner balance and tranquility, encourage elderly women to engage in this exercise and develop a deeper mind-body connection.

Closing: Take a few spontaneous breaths while keeping both nostrils open to complete the alternate nostril breathing exercise. Reposition your hands gently onto your thighs or lap, keeping your inner peace and stillness intact.

By incorporating Alternate Nostril Breathing with chair yoga, older women can benefit from a straightforward yet effective tool for overall wellbeing, mental clarity, and relaxation. Promote consistent use, incorporating this method into their daily regimen for a comprehensive approach to well-being.

Balance and Stability

For senior women over 60, balance and stability are essential components of chair yoga, since it not only enhances physical well-being but also boosts confidence and lowers the chance of falls. In the context of chair yoga, incorporating particular movements and mindfulness exercises can help to enhance stability and balance.

1. Seated Mountain Pose: To start, take a comfortable seat in the chair, plant your feet firmly, and extend your spine. A seated mountain posture is a stable stance. Connect with the chair's support and concentrate on a solid base.

 2. Weight Shifts: While seated, gently move your weight forward, backward,

and side to side. These small motions strengthen proprioception and work the core muscles, which promote balance and body awareness.

3. Seated Leg Lifts: Take a few deep breaths and raise one leg at a time, stretching it straight in front of you. This exercise enhances balance and fortifies the hip musculature. On both sides, repeat.

4. Ankle Rolls and Toe Taps: Perform ankle rolls and toe taps to improve stability and circulation. The muscles in the legs and feet are also used during these seated motions.

5. Chair Squats: Gently rise from the chair, leaning on it if necessary, and then take a seat again. Chair squats enhance stability and strengthen the

lower body. Increase the squat depth gradually as your strength increases.

6. Seated Side Stretch: Lean slightly to the side while seated and extend one arm above. This side stretch while seated works the lateral and core muscles, which enhances stability. On both sides, repeat.

7. Mindful Walking in Place: Try walking mindfully in place while clinging to the chair for stability. Lift your knees and plant your feet consciously to activate your leg muscles and improve your coordination.

8. Seated Tree Pose: While seated, raise one foot and plant it on the calf or inner thigh of the other leg. This modified tree makes it difficult to

maintain stability and balance while seated.

9. Seated Rotate with Arm Reach: Sitting upright, gently rotate your torso on one side while reaching across your body with your arm. Rotational stability is enhanced and the core is engaged in this movement. On both sides, repeat.

10. Mindful Breath Awareness: Stress the value of mindful breath awareness during these exercises for stability and balance. Motivate elderly women to align their breathing with their activities in order to promote focus and ease.

Closing:

After a brief period of seated silence, let participants consider how they felt about their stability and balance. Stress the benefits of consistent chair yoga practice for stronger muscles, better balance, and an overall sense of well-being.

By including these balance and stability exercises in chair yoga, senior women can progressively increase their strength, which boosts their self-esteem and lowers their chance of falling. Regular practice builds a stable feeling of awareness in daily tasks by establishing a mindful link between the body and mind.

Seated Leg Lifts

Chair yoga requires seated leg lifts, which are crucial for older ladies over sixty. They offer a gentle yet effective way to improve overall mobility, strengthen the lower body, and increase flexibility. Here's a comprehensive guide to introducing sitting leg lifts into your chair yoga practice:

Beginning Position: Sit comfortably in the chair, ensure your feet are firmly on the ground, and keep your back straight. Put your hands on your lap or on your thighs to create a comfortable and relaxed pose.

Take slow, deep breaths via your nose and out of your mouth while you engage in attentive awareness. To cultivate mindfulness, practice being fully present in each moment.

Step 1: Start by raising your right leg. Breathe deeply as you extend your right leg out in front of you.

2. Contract your quadriceps and feel the stretch in the back of your leg while you hold the elevated posture for a few breaths.

3. Breathe out as you progressively lower your right leg back to the floor.

Changing Sides: Perform the identical movements with your left leg, breathing in as you raise it, holding it for a short while, and then exhaling as you bring it back down. Keep your movements steady and fluid the entire time.

Some advice on seated leg lifts:

1. Engage Core Muscles: To stabilize and support your lower back during the leg lift, engage your core muscles.

2. Mindful Breathing: Align your movements and breathing. Breathe in as you raise your leg and out as you bring it down. The mind-body link is strengthened by this synchronization.

3. Comfortable Range: Raise your leg to a reasonable and comfortable height. Maintaining good form is more crucial than raising the leg excessively.

4. Repeat: Complete many rounds of the sequence for both legs, progressively increasing the number of repetitions as your comfort and strength allow.

The advantages of sitting leg lifts

1. Builds Quadriceps Strength: By focusing on the quadriceps, seated leg lifts help to strengthen the muscles in the front of the thighs.

2. Enhances Leg Flexibility: The raising motion aids in enhancing the back of the leg and hip flexors' flexibility.

3. Improves Circulation: Blood circulation is improved by elevating the leg, which is advantageous for vascular health in general.

4. Strengthens Mind-Body Connection: By encouraging a sense of awareness and present, the purposeful and focused character of seated leg lifts strengthens the mind-body connection.

Closing:

Let both feet rest on the ground to complete the seated leg lifts. Spend a few moments in silence, taking deep breaths, and noticing how your legs feel. Stress the benefits of constant practice on leg strength and flexibility, as well as the progressive growth.

Senior women who practice chair yoga with seated leg lifts are better able to maintain and strengthen their lower body, which enhances their general mobility and well-being. Through encouraging a mindful approach to movement, the practice builds body awareness and a sense of vigor.

Heel and Toe Taps

Heel and toe taps can be used in chair yoga for older ladies over 60 to help with circulation and flexibility. This is a mild workout where you sit and alternately tap the toe and heel of each foot. By engaging the lower extremities and preserving range of motion, these deliberate movements improve joint mobility.

Heel taps are a simple exercise that strengthens the muscles in the lower leg and encourages ankle flexibility by extending one leg forward and lightly tapping the heel on the ground. Seniors can benefit most from this exercise, as it improves balance and eases ankle stiffness.

Similar to this, toe taps entail raising the toes off the ground in order to strengthen the foot muscles and increase ankle joint flexibility. This is a useful exercise for reducing pain and increasing general foot mobility.

Chair yoga incorporates heel and toe taps into a low-impact exercise that is appropriate for senior citizens and helps them maintain a healthy range of motion in their lower limbs. For older women over 60, regular practice can help with decreased stiffness, increased circulation, and general well-being.

Flexibility Exercises

Flexibility exercises are essential for increasing joint mobility and reducing muscular tension in chair yoga for older ladies over 60. Flexibility can be increased with controlled, gentle motions that don't overstress the body.

Begin by teaching elders to rotate their necks slowly in both circular and sideways motions. This encourages flexibility and relieves stiffness by easing tension in the shoulders and neck.

Subsequently, you might use mild arm circles and shoulder rolls as shoulder stretches. These exercises reduce the pain associated with stiffness and help maintain the shoulder joints' flexibility.Sitting spinal twists are beneficial to the flexibility of the spine. It is important to teach seniors to sit up straight and to carefully rotate their upper bodies to one side, then the other. This promotes more spinal flexibility and helps to maintain a healthy range of motion.

Leg stretches while seated can be introduced for the lower body. To promote ankle flexibility, extend one leg at a time, flexing and pointing the foot. It is also possible to integrate mild knee lifts, which help to keep the knee joints flexible.

Finally, movements that involve toe pointing and ankle rotations help to increase the lower extremities' flexibility. Seniors benefit most from these activities because they improve circulation and help avoid foot and ankle stiffness.

By adding these stretches to chair yoga for elderly women over 60, you may support joint health and general flexibility in a gentle and approachable way, all while fostering a holistic approach to well-being. Frequent exercise can help with reduced stiffness, enhanced comfort in daily activities, and a greater range of motion.

Seated Leg Stretches

For older ladies over 60, chair yoga's seated leg stretches offer significant advantages. These mild stretches aid with lower body stress relief, circulation enhancement, and flexibility improvement. Start by placing your feet firmly on the floor and sitting comfortably in a sturdy chair. Flex your foot and extend one leg forward, keeping it straight but not locked.

Feel a stretch along the back of your leg as you gently bend forward from your hips. After a few breaths of holding, move to the opposite leg. Making a figure-four shape by crossing one ankle over the other knee is another useful stretch. Feel the stretch in your outer hip as you softly press down on the lifted knee while maintaining a straight back. Continue on the opposite side. These leg stretches while seated increase range of motion and can be easily added to an elder chair yoga practice to benefit general health in women.

Ankle Rolls

For senior ladies over 60, chair yoga's ankle rolls are a great way to increase ankle flexibility and improve circulation. First, take a comfortable seat in a chair and place your feet flat on the ground. With the heel still firmly planted, raise one foot just a little. Turn your ankle clockwise and then counterclockwise in a circular manner. This mild motion increases the range of motion and lubricates the ankle joint. Repeat the circular movements with the other ankle. Regular ankle rolls can help to keep joints healthy, lessen stiffness, and avoid the pain that comes with being immobile. This easy-to-learn chair yoga technique promotes flexibility in a comfortable seated position, which benefits elderly women's general well-being.

Cool Down and Relaxation

The goal of chair yoga for senior ladies over 60 is to unwind and calm down; it's a tranquil approach to wrapping up an exercise session. Sit comfortably in the chair and maintain a comfortable posture as you wind down. Breathe deeply and slowly to begin the relaxing process. Inhale deeply through your nose to fill your lungs with air, and then release any remaining tension by softly exhaling through your mouth.

Go on to mild neck stretches, slowly rotating your head in circles and tilting it from side to side. This helps to relieve tension that has built up in the shoulders and neck throughout the session. Maintain your seated forward bends, letting your upper body fall elegantly over your legs. This promotes flexibility by creating a small stretch along the spine.

Stretch your wrists and shoulders gently, paying attention to your movements. The purpose of these motions is to improve general comfort by releasing any remaining stiffness in these places. Ascend gradually to a calm condition that invites a quick mindfulness or meditation session. Shut your eyes, concentrate on your breathing, and release any residual thoughts.

Designed specifically for older women, this chair yoga cool-down and relaxation routine promotes physical ease and a calm state of mind. It acts as a soothing wrap-up for the practice, bringing participants' sensations of renewal and serenity.

Guided Relaxation

A number of soothing and gentle practices are used in chair yoga for elderly ladies over 60 to facilitate guided relaxation, lower stress levels, and improve general well-being. Below is a further explanation of this practice:

1. Comfortable Seating: First, make sure the elderly ladies are situated in supportive, firm chairs. This is vital to prevent any discomfort throughout the relaxing period.

2. Mindful Breathing: Concentrate on mindful breathing at first. Give participants instructions to breathe slowly and deeply, focusing on the significance of breathing via the nose and expelling through the mouth. In

doing so, the body's relaxation reaction is aided.

3. Body Scan: Lead them through a mild body scan, highlighting various body parts. To help them become more aware and relaxed, encourage them to identify any tension they may be feeling and to intentionally release it.

4. Visualization: Explain visualization methods and help them picture calm, quiet environments. This could be a garden, a beach, or any other location that inspires sentiments of peace. Urge them to visualize this with all of their senses.

5. Progressive Muscle Relaxation: Guide the elderly in tensing and then releasing various muscle areas through progressive muscle relaxation. This

increases the sensation of general relaxation and relieves physical stress.

6. Affirmations and Positive Imagery: To improve their mental health, use affirmations and positive imagery. Urge them to concentrate on affirmations that deal with acceptance, thankfulness, and self-compassion.

7. Gentle Movement: Include calming, flowing motions in your relaxation routine. Simple stretches, shoulder and neck motions, and wrist rotations are a few examples of them. The intention is to reduce tension and encourage flexibility.

8. Calm Music or Nature Noises: Put some calming music on repeat or play some natural noises to create a calm mood. This makes the whole experience

better and creates a more relaxing atmosphere.

9. Guided Meditation: Conduct a brief guided meditation with the group, concentrating on mindfulness or a particular subject like appreciation or loving-kindness. This may intensify your feeling of calmness and relaxation within.

10. Conclude the guided relaxation with a quick reflection that gives participants a chance to talk about their experiences and let out any emotions that may have come up. This promotes a feeling of solidarity and community.

To make the guided relaxation accessible, pleasurable, and advantageous for the senior women's general well-being, don't forget to adjust it to their own needs and talents.

Mindful Breathing

A key technique in chair yoga for elderly ladies over 60 is mindful breathing, which lowers stress, increases awareness, and promotes relaxation. For this group, here's a detailed tutorial on adding mindful breathing to chair yoga sessions:

1. Seated Posture: Let's start by stressing how important it is to sit comfortably and erect. Seniors should be urged to sit with their feet flat on the ground, shoulders relaxed, and backs straight. This guarantees the best possible alignment and support for attentive breathing.

2. Breath Awareness: Help people learn to be aware of their breathing. Stress the importance of your breathing's

natural rhythm and how it helps you stay in the present. Tell them to focus on the sensation of their breath coming into and going out of their bodies. 3. Nasal Breathing: Emphasize the significance of breathing through your nose. Nasal breathing also improves humidity and air quality and has several other physiological benefits, such as lowering nervous system activity.

4. Deep Belly Breaths: Start with deep belly breathing as a foundational technique. Tell them to expand their stomachs, take a deep breath through their noses, and then gently release it through their lips to release any tension. This diaphragmatic breathing promotes relaxation and reduces stress.

5. Counted Breaths: Use a counting method to help you concentrate. Help them count each breath, up to maybe five, and then restart. This easy-to-count exercise reduces distractions and helps you stay focused.

6. Mindful Observation: Promote observing the breath mindfully without trying to change it. Remind participants that accepting and observing the breath rather than trying to alter it is the aim. This fosters an awareness of the current moment that is free from judgment.

7. Breath Awareness with Movement: Combine mindful breathing with mild motions. As an example, assist them in raising their arms during inhalation and lowering them during exhalation. This breathing and movement coordination

cultivates flow and improves consciousness.

8. Guided Imagery with Breath: This technique combines guided imagery with conscious breathing. Encourage participants to imagine breathing in a calming hue or positive energy and to imagine releasing any tension or stress when they exhale. This gives the activity a creative and calming element.

9. Breath Awareness Meditation: Include a seated breath awareness meditation during a segment of the chair yoga practice. As you lead them through a prolonged period of breath awareness, let the thoughts come and go without attachment. This fosters consciousness on a deeper level.

10. Closing Reflection: Give a quick reflection to wrap up the mindful breathing exercise. Invite people to talk about their experiences or any realizations they had while practicing. This creates a chance for interaction and highlights the good of deliberate breathing.

Chair yoga sessions for senior women over 60 can benefit from the use of mindful breathing, as it lays the groundwork for improved well-being, reduced stress, and increased present-moment awareness. Make sure each participant has a safe and pleasurable experience by customizing the practices to meet their unique requirements and interests.

Conclusion

Finally, chair yoga becomes apparent as a comprehensive and approachable wellness technique designed especially for senior women sixty years of age and older. In addition to meeting this population's physical demands, this low-impact yet effective exercise also tends to their mental and emotional well. Chair yoga offers a comprehensive method of improving general health through a deliberate fusion of sitting postures, focused breathing, mild movements, and guided relaxation.

No matter their level of fitness or mobility restrictions, participants can engage in the practice safely thanks to the emphasis on correct alignment, adaptability, and steady advancement. The foundation is the application of mindful breathing, which promotes presence, peace, and self-awareness. This helps elders, in particular, by reducing stress and fostering a link between the body and mind.

Furthermore, chair yoga extends beyond the area of physical exercise into the community and emotional support domains. The senior women's sense of belonging and camaraderie is fostered by the social contract that is encouraged in the group environment. In addition to fostering physical wellness, the common practice of movement and mindfulness also fosters an upbeat and happy attitude.

Chair yoga is a technique that empowers older women by being flexible and enabling them to accept and cherish their bodies at any stage of life. It reminds us that wellbeing is a journey and that each participant's needs and talents are catered to in this practice. Senior women over 60 who practice chair yoga start a journey of self-care that extends beyond their physical well-being and includes mental clarity, emotional resilience, and a community of support.

Chair yoga ultimately serves as evidence for the idea that enjoying a happy and healthy lifestyle may happen at any age. It provides an environment where older women may take care of their health, practice mindfulness, and embrace their inner energy. Chair yoga unfolds as a gift—an invitation to embrace life's richness with grace and vitality—as a holistic and inclusive practice.